SHEILA ZIMMERMANN

Tips from a Castor Oil Enthusiast

Discover the Beauty and Health Benefits at your fingertips

Copyright © 2024 by Sheila Zimmermann

All rights reserved. No part of this publication may be reproduced, stored or transmitted in any form or by any means, electronic, mechanical, photocopying, recording, scanning, or otherwise without written permission from the publisher. It is illegal to copy this book, post it to a website, or distribute it by any other means without permission.

Sheila Zimmermann asserts the moral right to be identified as the author of this work.

Sheila Zimmermann has no responsibility for the persistence or accuracy of URLs for external or third-party Internet Websites referred to in this publication and does not guarantee that any content on such Websites is, or will remain, accurate or appropriate.

Designations used by companies to distinguish their products are often claimed as trademarks. All brand names and product names used in this book and on its cover are trade names, service marks, trademarks and registered trademarks of their respective owners. The publishers and the book are not associated with any product or vendor mentioned in this book. None of the companies referenced within the book have endorsed the book.

First edition

This book was professionally typeset on Reedsy.
Find out more at reedsy.com

Contents

1

Introduction

Welcome to the Tips from a Castor Oil Enthusiast. My name is Sheila Zimmermann and I am very excited to write this book. A Castor Oil enthusiast? What is THAT you might ask? It sounds funny even to me. Why write about Castor Oil? To be clear from the start - I am not a health expert and am certainly not here to give you medical advice.

My purpose for writing this book is to share with you the bits of knowledge that I have discovered and used with regards to Castor Oil.

I find that deep down we are all a "health expert" for ourselves and our body and perhaps this extends to our family - spouse, children and loved ones including our furry family members. We know intuitively what works and what doesn't and the more we trust ourselves the better life progresses.

A brief background - I have had and continue to have a happy and fulfilling life with a Music career as a professional Flutist alongside my husband and Pianist, Eric Zimmermann. We have raised two beautiful children and have enjoyed the company of our many cat companions.

Throughout the years I have tended to lean towards natural and holistic solutions for health, addressing things as they emerged and have kept busy living life. But as I grow older I find that I have attention and concern in some personal areas - my skin, a few aches here and there, digestive issues, etc. Nothing major - but they steal my attention away from life and livingness. So I found myself searching here and there for solutions.

To my delight Castor Oil has recently exploded onto the information highway as a natural remedy for many health and beauty issues. Castor Oil? Wasn't that something the midwife suggested to use if one wished to go into labor? Or some mysterious liquid given to children way back in my parents and grandparents day?

I am so happy to have stumbled upon Castor Oil and my hope is that the tips that I have provided in these following pages can help you with those "attention stealers" so that you can address them and bring verve and joy back into your life. And who knows, you might become a Castor Oil enthusiast yourself!

Happy reading and happy living!

2

Castor Oil Basics

What is Castor Oil

Castor Oil is a colorless or pale yellow oil that is extracted from the seed of the Castor plant, known scientifically as Ricinus communis. The plants are native to the Ethiopian region of East Africa but India produces the bulk of Castor Oil as well as China and Brazil topping the list of exporters.

For the best quality of oil one should purchase only cold pressed Castor Oil and it should be stored in a dark glass container. It is not advisable to purchase it in a plastic container since the oil can break down the plastic bottle.

Also the oil should be Hexane free as Hexane is an organic compound used to extract oils from seeds and is toxic to humans and can cause allergic reactions.

Links for Castor Oils can be found at the end under Products and Links

Castor Oil has blossomed as a solution for a variety of uses and ailments.. One of the main reasons for this is that Castor oil is rich in Ricinoleic Acid, a type of fatty acid that has anti-inflammatory and antioxidant properties. Because of this Castor Oil can be found in a variety of uses in both Beauty and Health.

History of Castor Oil

Castor Oil has been found in Egyptian tombs dating back to 4,000 B.C. Cleopatra used Castor Oil to maintain her beauty and even added it to her eyes to make them appear brighter. It has also been used in Ayurvedic medicine (a traditional Hindu medicine) for digestion and detoxification and in Chinese Medicine for its anti-inflammatory properties as well as to relieve pain.

Castor Oil was a main health staple in Africa as a hair treatment as well as for the scalp, skin and body. Castor beans were brought to America by Africans in the late 1600's and were used as a medicinal property.

One of the main uses of Castor Oil and the only approved use by the FDA is for its laxative properties to relieve temporary constipation.

The only time I had heard about Castor Oil was for use in inducing labor as well as being spoon-fed to children for various unknown ailments. Somehow in all my years I never came across the amazing health benefits of Castor Oil until only a short time ago.

Suffice it to say that pregnant women should avoid Castor Oil or consult their Doctor or Midwife regarding its use during pregnancy.

3

Beauty Benefits

C**astor Oil - Skin Deep
About Face**

Castor Oil first caught my attention when I saw a YouTube Video outlining the benefits on the skin - particularly the face. Unfortunately facial lines and wrinkles are a part of life and I, like many others, have searched high and low as well as spent countless dollars chasing the perfect skin solution. Most cosmetic lines sell special creams and serums promising a reduction in fine lines around the eyes, forehead and mouth.

So my first video that I saw on Castor oil was by Shea Whitney entitled "I Used CASTOR OIL for 30 Days and THIS Happened!!!" I have to say that her ENTHUSIASM was infectious. Within 30 minutes I went from mildly curious to strongly determined to try Castor Oil - going to Amazon and ordering the recommended type in a dark glass container.

(See link below for her video)

I loved that she explained the benefits and tips for the body from the top (the head - hair and face) to the bottom (feet). I was particularly intrigued by the tips for the face. So when I got my Castor Oil about 45 days ago I began using it morning and night particularly on my face.

Note:
   I have attached a link to this video and all other videos mentioned. You can find them at the end of the book under "Products and Video Links".

Before using Castor Oil I found that my face would tend to be reddish in the morning with dark circles and sometimes I would have puffiness under the eyes depending on how much sleep or more precisely - the lack of sleep - that I had the night before. Also I tended to have large pores, particularly around my nose area mostly due to having oily skin and acne when I was younger. I found that my pores tended to be clogged easily with the various makeups and concealers that I have used throughout the years and every once in a while I would get a small breakout even at my age. But after using Castor Oil for about 45 days I find that my pores have gotten significantly smaller and my skin is not oily but instead it is soft and moist. Castor oil is thick and at first I thought "I cannot put this on my face as it will definitely cause problems and clog my pores and make my skin more oily". But on the contrary I found that it was such an amazing and natural moisturizer and that my skin seemed to absorb it fully. It was so different from any other moisturizer that I have used in the past that I will never go back.

The redness that I experienced on a regular basis is practically gone and the dark circles under my eyes are greatly reduced. I still find that they appear when I lose sleep but it has drastically improved. It has been said by Shea and others that Castor Oil is Nature's Botox and I wholeheartedly and enthusiastically agree!!

Also stated in her video is that Castor Oil has so many powerful properties. It is loaded with minerals and 18 Fatty Acids including Omega 6's and 9's as well as Vitamin E. As a result Castor OIl with its antioxidant properties goes to work against free radicals on the skin and helps to reduce fine lines and wrinkles.

Another Video by a Castor Oil enthusiast Solar Girl Homestead mentioned that Castor Oil is such a great moisturizer because it is really good at locking in moisture and also it helps to pull moisture into the skin from the environment and air.

Castor Oil is great to use alone. But you can also combine it with your favorite moisturizer or skin product and the Castor Oil will enhance the performance of that moisturizer or skin cream.

I found two videos that gave tips on how to increase the benefits of Castor Oil by Three Times:

The first is, again, by Solar Girl Homestead. She has created a natural moisturizer using rice water, aloe vera and flaxseed gel. Castor Oil will enhance this natural moisturizer and increase the benefits to your skin by three times.

The second video is by Patty - Sixty is the New Sixty. For a face massage she combines ½ Castor Oil with ½ Rosehip Oil and 8 drops of Frankincense into a 2 oz. bottle. She has also tried Sesame Oil as a substitute for Rosehip Oil. Patty also discusses Ice Water Dips for the

Face and she fully explains it in the video below.

Facial Massage

Another great use for Castor Oil is for massaging the face. One can use what is called a Gua Sha Stone, an ancient Chinese method of scraping the skin with a special stone, usually made of Jade or Rose Quartz, to improve circulation and reduce inflammation. Using this technique with Castor Oil will help the oil penetrate into your skin and allow the anti-inflammatory and antioxidant properties to help fight free radicals and may slow the aging process.

I found this site to be really helpful in finding more information on Gua Sha stones including helpful tips for use in doing a facial massage.

Another great tip came from Castor Oil enthusiast Chalene Johnson. In her video she said that sometimes you don't have a Gua Sha stone available with you. But you always have your knuckles. She demonstrates a great lymphatic massage that she does along the jawline that I have incorporated since using Castor Oil.

Charlene states that using this massage for over a year has definitely changed her jawline and that she can see results in pictures side by side. Basically you take your knuckles and place them on your chin and massage out toward your ears and then down the sides of the neck and repeat up to 10 times or more. It is an easy addition to your morning or night cleansing routine and I have noticed improvement in the definition of my jawline. She also massages from the top of the bridge of the nose down the nose and then under the cheekbones and continues out to the temples repeating this 10 - 15 times.

The Face & Acne

Castor Oil is great for Acne prone skin since it is antimicrobial and anti-inflammatory. The Ricinoleic Acid found in Castor Oil inhibits the growth of acne-causing bacteria and helps to reduce the redness and irritation that occurs in acne breakouts.

In researching Castor oil and Acne I came across this video where Sonia Anastasia used Castor Oil on her face for two weeks and I saw the improvement in her skin and the effective results on her acne. She said many times in the video how the Castor Oil made her skin feel moisturized and smooth. Here is the link below so you can watch her two week progression:

Castor Oil Packs for Acne

Another effective way to help with Acne is to detoxify one's liver with a Castor Oil Pack. Castor Oil Packs were first invented by Edgar Cayce (1877 - 1945) who used them to help with many symptoms. Basically A Castor Oil Pack is the use of material, either cotton or flannel soaked with Castor Oil and placed on the area that one wishes to address. Some use heating pads or a hot water bottle to heat the area. The video below has great tips for using Castor Oil to detoxify the liver with a Castor Oil Pack. Dr. Stacey Shillington ND goes into great detail in the video below on how Castor Oil helps with the lymph system to help detoxify your liver and help clear up acne. Also below is a link for the Castor Oil Pack that she recommends.

Sunburns, Rashes, etc.

Sunburns can be so painful and I tend to burn easily due to my Irish heritage. I am mindful about using sunscreen and have used Aloe Vera in the past to calm my sunburns. I am excited to hear that Castor Oil can help soothe the pain connected with sunburn due to its anti-inflammatory properties. Also the Ricinoleic Acid helps with blistering and peeling of the skin. One can use both Aloe Vera as well as Castor oil to speed up the healing of sunburn and I intend to incorporate Castor Oil in my Sunburn fighting arsenal.

Rashes happen. I sometimes get a rash from an insect bite where I scratch too much. Recently this occurred on my arm and I put Castor oil on the rash and it was gone within 24 hours.

Another Castor Oil Enthusiast Sally Atkins with her channel Fabulous over 50 discussed all of her benefits from using Castor Oil for 30 days and what struck me the most was her success with handling various rashes and redness that she would experience. She began putting Castor Oil on her skin at the onset of a rash or redness or allergic reaction and it completely handled it, most likely due to the anti-inflammatory properties.

She also mentioned that Castor Oil helped with pigmentation of her sun damaged skin and age spots on the hands due most likely to the high Vitamin E content in Castor Oil.

But the most amazing one on her video was that she used Castor Oil on a Keloid Scar. (A Keloid Scar is a scar that occurs due to a surgical incision or a scar with excessive tissue). She had one of these scars from a mosquito bite which created a lump on her skin. She put Castor Oil on it and it shrunk to half it's size. She was so thrilled!

It is so amazing to me how many ways that Castor Oil can help with skin issues.

Another Castor Oil Enthusiast, Melissa Gallagher, a Natural Doctor, Nutritionist & Lymphatic Drainage Therapist, mentioned using Castor Oil Packs on Varicose and Spider Veins in her video listing 20 Surprising Benefits of Castor Oil Pack Therapy. The Castor Oil Pack helped to tighten the skin and ease the pain from the Varicose Vein that was affecting her leg.

Melissa also mentioned that Castor Oil is great for Eczema and Psoriasis as it has antibacterial properties and helps to alleviate these skin conditions by penetrating into the dermal layers and easing the inflammation.

Let's face it. Castor Oil is AMAZING for any skin condition. You name it - it can help with Stretch Marks, breaking up scar tissue as well as reducing cellulite. Maybe you will find some unique uses for Castor Oil for your skin. The great thing is that it is inexpensive, natural and toxic free. So take the plunge and experiment with Castor Oil on your skin - for beauty as well as for other skin conditions. And may your skin never be the same again.

4

Other Beauty Benefits

To Hair or Not to Hair
Hair Growth and Hair Care

One of the main topics addressed with regards to Castor Oil is its use in Hair Growth. Be it stress, aging or our ever increasing toxic world, hair loss is a current problem in our society today with many looking for help with this problem. As I researched this I found that there were so many Castor Oil enthusiasts reporting thicker hair while at the same time more traditional medical sites cautioned that "there is no scientific evidence to support hair growth from Castor Oil". While it is advisable not to make wild, medical claims - I find that the enthusiasm and the testimonials of so many people have encouraged me to "take the hair plunge" and try it out for myself.

Some tips: since it is a very thick oil - there are many ways to use it on the hair. You can add a few drops to your scalp, massage in and leave overnight and wash your hair in the morning.

13

I shared my Castor Oil enthusiasm with my dear friend Devorah and she found that using too much matted her hair down. So she decided to add some Castor Oil to her shampoo instead of applying it directly to her hair.

Also the shampoo she began using is by L'Oreal for Curly Hair and she discovered that it already has Castor Oil as one of the ingredients.

Using this shampoo and adding a bit of Castor Oil to it has been the ideal use for Devorah to create fuller, thicker and shinier hair.

Castor Oil is great for hair breakage as well as split ends. Place a small amount of Castor Oil onto your palms and rub on the ends of your hair or areas that seem weak and prone to breakage. Leave overnight and then wash out in the morning.

Years ago I would blow dry my hair nearly every day and it somehow could tolerate the heat. But these past few years I have found that my hair has changed. Despite using conditioners and allowing it to dry naturally I find that in general it looks dry and a bit frizzy and wild. Applying Castor Oil to the ends have really made quite a difference and I have noticed that my hair is smoother, shinier and less dry looking.

I look forward to trying some scalp treatments as well as adding Castor Oil to my shampoo as mentioned above.

Lashes and Brows

Once again the Castor Oil Enthusiasts score high marks when it comes to their lashes and brows. I have heard over and over from multiple sources that Castor Oil helps to grow thicker eyelashes and fuller eyebrows. But again, the medical sources caution that "there is no definitive scientific proof that Castor Oil promotes lash and brow growth".

Some people have short or small lashes as well as thin brows and as we age our lashes and brows get thinner. But who can argue with actual testimonial proof and excitement of longer lashes and thicker brows. Why not try it on the brows and brush some on the lashes. Or you can order small lash brushes and brush some on your lashes and see for yourself.

Nails and Cuticles

My hands and nails have it rough. I am not gentle with them nor do I use gloves when washing dishes, gardening or cleaning. As a result my hands, nails and especially my cuticles suffer. It has been a long standing problem for me. But since using Castor Oil on my face primarily, while applying it with my fingers, a side benefit occurred where I have less hangnails, my cuticles are a lot less dry and bothersome and my nails seem stronger and less pronc to breaking.

Castor Oil Enthusiast Shea Whitney made another great video entitled 15 New "Incredible Ways to Use Castor Oil:". In this video she mentions that you can purchase a small bottle with a roller top and put Castor Oil in there and then use it on your cuticles and nails to soften the cuticles and grow harder and stronger nails. I'm sure you can just take Castor Oil and apply it directly but I like the idea of the roller top bottle. It is super convenient to toss in your purse and have with you on the go. I find I am in my car a lot for work and so I can easily apply Castor Oil to my fingers while in traffic.

Lips

I really love applying Castor to my lips. Again while applying Castor Oil initially to my face it only seemed natural to apply some to my lips. I am so thrilled that my lips feel naturally soft and moist. I tend to not use any lip gloss or lipstick in general and I find that my lips get pretty dry throughout the day. But since using Castor Oil I love the feel of my lips and actually look forward to applying some lip gloss. Sally Atkins of Fabulous Over 50 remarks that her lip lines have diminished since using Castor Oil as a Lip Balm and she is so thrilled over this.

Natural Face Cleanser

Shea Whitney has shared a new tip for Castor Oil. One can use it as a Natural Face Cleanser. You add it to your dry skin to remove makeup and then follow up with washing your face as usual. I think this is brilliant as commercial makeup removers can have harsh chemicals added whereas this is a natural cleanser.

Also she suggests adding Castor Oil to your body gel that you use in the shower. When you are done your skin has had the benefit of being fully clean as well as moisturized. You can still add Castor Oil to your body as you desire, but I like the idea of getting the benefits while showering.

Tattoo Care

I was so happy to hear this tip from Shea Whitney. About a month ago my daughter & I designed and got matching tattoos - she got hers on the back of her right arm above the elbow and I got mine on the left arm in the same place. She had gotten a tattoo last year and was sharing her ideas for her second one. Her ideas and creativity piqued my interest and before I knew it we were scheduled to get our tattoos - flowers that represent each of us - roses for her and an Iris for me. Rose is my daughter's birth month flower (and her favorite flower) and my birth month flower is Lilies of the Valley. However - I love Irises and so that was the extent of my creativity. The rest came from my daughter. Needless to say I was nervous - what am I doing getting a tattoo? Isn't this just for younger folks? Then there was the pain factor - which I admit I felt very fearful about right up to the moment he started. I had to chuckle as I had mentally worked up such a fear about the pain - but in reality it was hardly painful at all.

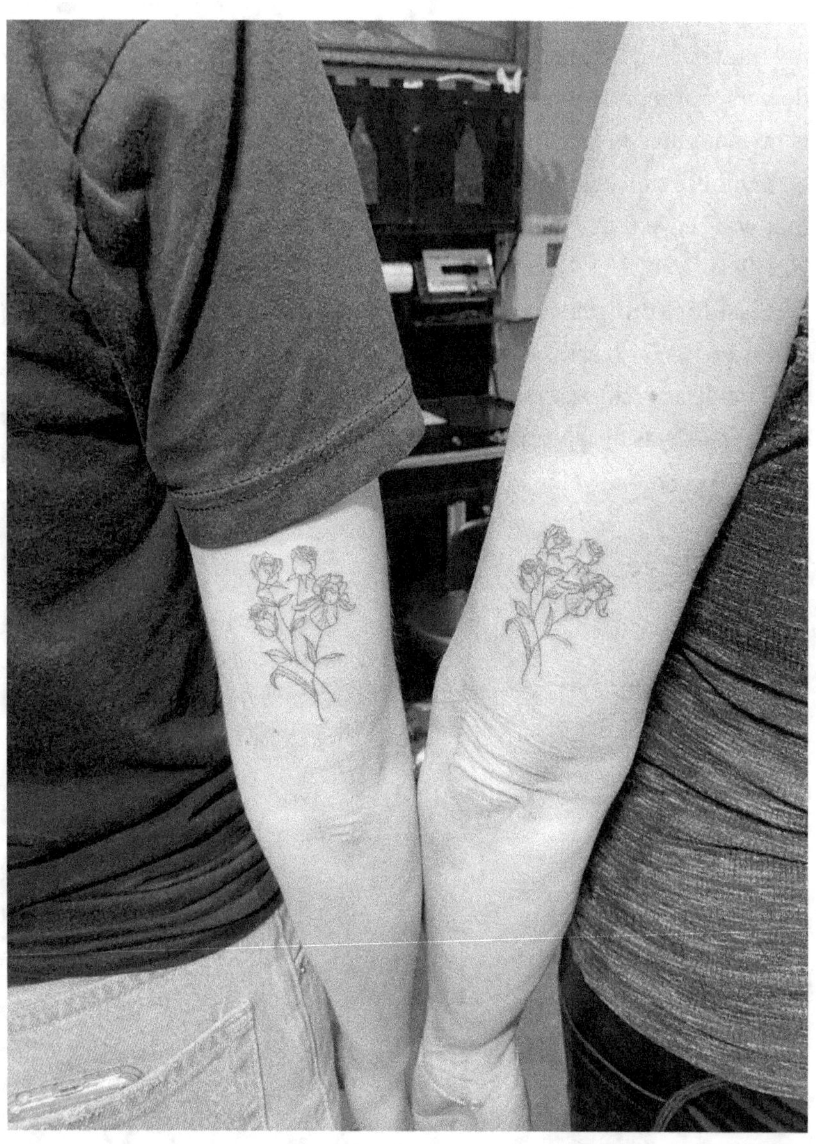

After the tattoo we got a care sheet. Once the bandage was removed, after a few days, we were to wash the tattoo with soap and water and then put lotion on it to keep it moist and help with the itchiness and peeling skin. He suggested a few lotions and I asked "what about Castor Oil?" He had a surprised look on his face, paused and then said that I shouldn't use Castor Oil. I asked this because I was at that time happily enjoying the benefits of Castor Oil on my face.

I was so delighted when I saw Shea Whitney's latest video offering Castor Oil for Tattoo Care. It will soothe the pain and redness of the tattoo on the skin and due to its antimicrobial and antibacterial properties it will help fight off possible infections. So intuitively I was right about using Castor Oil and now I can share this tip with the tattoo artist for when my daughter gets her next one (& perhaps mine as well).

5

Health Benefits

I am so excited to share the myriad of health benefits that Castor Oil provides. I have tried several listed below and can attest to the efficacy and miraculous benefits of Castor Oil to aid in those nagging and annoying health problems that steal attention and fun from life. My hope is that the tips below will help you in your quest for natural solutions to your health issues.

Digestion & Constipation
  Nature's Plumbing

There is nothing worse, in my opinion, than having digestive issues. Whether it is due to stress or eating the wrong foods or lack of sleep I find that digestive issues can turn a happy, productive day into a problematic nightmare.

Thank goodness for Castor Oil! Due to its Ricinoleic Acid content

Castor Oil has been hailed as Nature's Laxative. One can consume Castor Oil for this and perhaps this is the only way I knew about it when I was younger. But there are many other tips to help with digestion and constipation.

The Belly Button

In researching Castor Oil the most commonly used and talked about method involves one's Navel or Belly Button. The Umbilical Cord was the main source of all of the nutrition and oxygen that we received from our Mother as we were developing in the womb. After we are born the Umbilical Cord is cut and after healing we are left with the Umbilicus or the Belly Button. But there is also an inner side to the umbilical cord that contains veins and arteries that also dry up and harden and become ligaments that remain attached to the inside portion of the belly button. These ligaments connect to our liver as well as our pelvic area where they assist with circulatory functions.

Because of this knowledge I can really see why using Castor Oil with the belly button would create such amazing health benefits. One use is to massage or rub Castor Oil onto the abdomen at night and let it absorb into the skin to assist the intestines and colon with digestion and elimination. I have tried this method for about a month now and I am quite pleased with the results.

But a more common tip is to pour a small amount of Castor Oil into the Navel or Belly Button area and lie horizontally for 20 - 30 minutes and then wipe off. Many using this tip have found that they have more regular bowel movements and less bloating and constipation. Some are sensitive to this and experience extreme elimination. This is probably due to the fact that Castor Oil helps with detoxification due to its antioxidant and antimicrobial properties. You know your body best - so perhaps starting with a small amount or trying this only a few times a week as opposed to every day will yield better results.

Belly Fat

Who doesn't want to trim down and handle the dreaded belly fat that accumulates as we get older. I found a wonderful video by Dr. Janine Bowring ND where she uses Castor Oil to help melt this belly fat. I have recently discovered this and will be trying this over the next few weeks.

She describes this tip or hack fully in the video below - but to summarize - one massages Castor Oil all around the abdomen as well as the back (as that is where the kidneys are). She then massages the abdomen 5 times clockwise and also massages the Ileocecal valve for a bit and then finishes with making downward motions 5 times from the abdomen down to the pelvic area. Then she wraps a cotton or flannel cloth around the abdomen and holds it in place with a waist trainer and wears it overnight.

I am especially excited to try this as I have discovered for me that my ileocecal valve can really wreak havoc on my digestive health. About 5 - 6 years ago I recall waking up one morning with flu like symptoms - slight fever, sweaty, body aches as well as a headache and feeling overall very lethargic. At the time I visited my Chiropractor and he determined that my Ileocecal valve was stuck.

What is an ileocecal valve? Well - it is a valve that separates the small and large intestines. It is located near the appendix in the lower right side of the abdomen. Its main job is to open and close and move food through one's digestive tract. Unfortunately it can get stuck - stuck open or stuck closed. As my Chiropractor used to say "the trash compactor stops working and wreaks havoc on the plumbing (one's intestines)." He would make a simple adjustment and within hours the symptoms would subside.

Now I know when I get these symptoms what could be causing it and there are times when I just massage the ileocecal valve and all goes back to normal. I look forward to trying out this Castor Oil massage and wrap. According to Dr. Janine Bowring it can help to extract toxins, improve circulation and glutathione levels, help with estrogen detoxification (which contributes to belly fat) and above all else melt belly fat.

Pain Reduction and other Health Tips

One of the greatest natural benefits from Castor Oil is its ability to lessen pain and inflammation. Instead of relying solely on pain medications with its addictive qualities, toxicity and side effects, we can tackle pain naturally with Castor Oil. One can apply Castor Oil directly onto the skin or use Castor Oil Wraps and greatly reduce pain, inflammation and speed up recovery.

I learned so many tips from Castor Oil enthusiast Melissa Gallagher, a Natural Doctor, Nutritionist & Lymphatic Drainage Therapist. In her video she lists 20 benefits of Castor Oil Packs to help you take control and help relieve pain . I have listed a few here but have added her link to her video so you can watch it and get her information in full.

Here are a few areas that Castor Oil can help:

• Arthritis, joint pain and muscle soreness can be greatly reduced by wrapping the areas with a Castor Oil pack or by rubbing Castor Oil directly onto the skin.

• Back pain can be relieved - whether it is the upper or lower back. You can massage Castor Oil onto the affected muscles or apply Castor Oil packs to the affected areas. Also Sciatic pain can be relieved as well.

• Headaches. You can apply a Castor Oil pack to the back of your neck. Also you can rub some Castor Oil onto your temples, forehead or wherever the pain is.

• Menstrual Cramps can be alleviated by wrapping a Castor Oil pack around the abdomen and applying heat.

• Adrenals can get overworked and stressed and, according to Melissa, can cause a wired/tired feeling. Castor Oil packs placed on the adrenals or rubbed into the area will help you to relax and unwind and will promote better sleep.

- Wound healing after surgical procedures can be greatly improved with Castor Oil packs. The packs can help with lymph drainage, increase blood flow, reduce swelling and bruising and in the long run help with minimizing scarring production.

- Fertility issues, while not necessarily physically painful, can be emotionally draining. Castor Oil packs can help with cysts on ovaries, inflamed fibroid and fibrotic tissue and can help to balance the hormones and communication between the ovaries, fallopian tubes and uterus.

Eyes and Feet and Bumps, Oh My!

In my research I have come across many testimonials from Castor Oil Enthusiasts regarding some pretty surprising benefits. I will share a few here.

- Shea Whitney had a callous on her pinkie toe that she developed from wearing ill-fitting shoes. She had the callous for 15 years and it was red and bothersome. She applied some Castor Oil on a bandage and placed it on the Callous and after a week and a half the callous was greatly reduced and the redness was completely gone..

- Shea also used a few drops of Castor Oil in a humidifier and placed it in her son's room. He had a stuffy nose and the next day he could breathe easier and felt much better.

• Dr. Kim D'Eramo did backcountry skiing years earlier and was ill-fitted for AT (All Terrain) Boots. The boots caused a bump/nodule on her foot below her pinkie toe and another bump on the right side of the other foot. She decided to put Castor Oil on them and noticed that they shrank in size.

• Dr. Kim also has had a nodule on her ear (also known as telephone operator's ear) for a few years. It started to hurt her while she was sleeping and so she consulted a friend/plastic surgeon. They told her that it is a callous and can be surgically removed or that she can sleep on a foam pillow to not put pressure on it. But… after using Castor Oil on it for a few weeks it is not totally gone but it is getting smaller and the best part is that there is no more pain.

• Castor Oil's benefits for the eyes includes reducing dry eyes as well as addressing floaters. The usual way of using it is to put a small amount on the eyelids.

• Liz with Stylish and Grateful - Fashion over 40 shared a great testimonial regarding her eyes and vision. She finds that her night vision is really poor and sometimes she has to go from working on the computer to a very dark room.. Usually she cannot see anything, not even inches from her face. But one day, after using Castor Oil for a bit of time, she walked into a dark room in her house and she could see. Not perfectly or clearly but it was a marked improvement.

6

Beyond the Body

Interesting Castor Oil Tips

Shea Whitney's recent Castor Oil video shared some amazing tips that are so clever and helpful. Here are a few of them:

- Cats are great groomers. But they end up with hairballs and that is no fun for anyone. Luckily Castor Oil comes in handy to help with this. You can add a few drops into their food. Start out small as cats can get pretty finicky with any changes. The Castor Oil will help with their digestion and the battle of the hairballs will lessen.

- Castor Oil can be a great replacement for WD 40 All Purpose Lubricant. Do you have a squeaky door hinge? Well - simply put some Castor Oil on a paper towel, apply to the hinge and voila - no more squeaks.

- Castor Oil is a great conditioner for leather shoes and handbags. Applying the oil leaves your leather items shiny and supple.

- Is your outdoor furniture or some metal item suffering from rust? Well - Castor Oil can help. Add a generous amount to the rust spots and let sit overnight. Then take a dry bristle brush and scrub the rust away. Your lawn furniture will thank you and you will be ready for your next outdoor party.

- Speaking of summer - Castor oil is a great natural insect repellent. You can ditch those toxic commercial products and apply Castor Oil to the skin and it will ward away mosquitos and other unwanted insects.

- Plants can suffer from unwanted insects and Castor Oil can help. Just mix equal parts of Castor Oil, water and dish soap into a spray bottle and apply to your garden and your plants will breathe a sigh of relief. This is a win win as you can then enjoy insect free vegetables and herbs.

7

Conclusion

I hope you have enjoyed reading Tips from a Castor Oil Enthusiast as much as I have enjoyed creating this book . I cannot help to get enthused and excited about sharing what I know to help bring about solutions to others.

Perhaps you are starting to get more interested in Castor Oil and have learned about a tip or two. My hope is that I was able to help you with some nagging issue or relieve some pains and discomforts that you might have. Or possibly piqued your interest in trying Castor Oil in ways you never could have imagined.

If you found this book helpful, I would very much appreciate it if you could leave a favorable review for the book on Amazon.

8

Products and Video Links

Castor Oils on Amazon

- RejuveNaturals Castor Oil (16oz Glass Bottle) USDA Certified Organic, 100% Pure, Cold Pressed, Hexane Free. Boost Hair Growth for Thicker, Fuller Hair, Lashes & Eyebrows.
  - https://a.co/d/gfOlqf8

- J MAC BOTANICALS, Organic Castor Oil Cold Pressed (Glass Bottle, 16 oz) pure unrefined,hexane free for face, skin, eyelashes, pack wraps, pads
- https://a.co/d/ehYyZiY

- QUEEN OF THE THRONES Organic Golden Castor Oil - 500mL (16.9oz) | 100% Pure & Expeller-Pressed for Hair, Skin & Digestion | Hexane Free | USDA Certified
- https://a.co/d/6HSmfcv

- Heritage Store Organic Castor, Glass Bottle, Cold Pressed, Rich Hydration for Hair & Skin, Bold Lashes & Brows | 16oz
- https://a.co/d/aN4NVEf

Video Links - About Face

Shea Whitney I Used CASTOR OIL for 30 Days and THIS Happened!!!
https://youtu.be/t1r72bbfG10?si=WU-UjvNpR8kqKWEu

Solar Girl Homestead Castor Oil For Your Face | INCREASE benefits by 3 TIMES | The Right WAY to use it to
https://youtu.be/U4tYTUxXPwQ?si=o_4GFHI6sqBWHFr-

Solar Girl Homestead
The Best Moisturizer: Removes Wrinkles, Scars, and gives Amazing Complexion
https://youtu.be/NaVP7v5rM9Q?si=Vq6KhSfZ2V1EUvHc

Patty - Sixty is the New 60 Turbo Charge Your Castor Oil and Face Massage with Ice Water Dips Over 50
https://youtu.be/ZRmpixiQ5Kc?si=VtJ2G9h-1dYp7jCk

Video Links - Facial Massage

What Is Gua Sha, and How Do You Use It to Sculpt Your Skin? Written by Lisa Marie Basile, MFA | Reviewed by Maria Robinson, MD, MBAhttps://www.goodrx.com/well-being/alternative-treatments/gua-sha-facial-stone-benefits

Chalene Johnson
Castor Oil Changed My Skin in 30 Days (SHOCKING RESULTS Over 50)
https://youtu.be/rXvD2e_FLhc?si=09Msd0Vm99hJXT8v

Video Links - The Face and Acne

Sonia Anastasia I TESTED PURE CASTOR OIL ON MY FACE FOR MY ACNE SCARS FOR 2 WEEKS || My review and thoughts!
https://youtu.be/J-jG2ZsqrG8?si=AbBebWgP1csRqbSs

Video Links - Castor Oil Packs for Acne

Dr. Stacey Shillington ND Naturopathic Beauty How Castor Oil Can Get Rid of your Acne
https://youtu.be/cK2wYh6a9Nk?si=KLWUCVB-UCnRKUtH

- Abdominal Castor Oil Pack Kit + Organic Castor Oil 16.9oz https://shopdrmarisol.com/collections/us-store/products/cast or-oil-pack-and-500ml-oil-bundle?cookieUUID=3cf19712-44f5-4f5b-acc5-87310280f806&cookieUUID=6309479d-0d57-4b85-a 029-e2b131d7c551&affiliate=284

Video Links - Sunburns, Rashes, etc.

Sally Atkins My SHOCKING Castor Oil Results After 30 Days As a Woman Over 50 Fabulous over 50
https://youtu.be/mhg86xl8v5Q?si=uC5WkJELeWRKDI_9

Melissa Gallagher 20 SURPRISING Benefits of Castor Oil Pack Therapy | Castor Oil Uses for Wellness
https://youtu.be/Kl9Z4d0R6hw?si=HlzDq-w9tVTWOz7X

Products and Video Links - Other Beauty Benefits Hair Growth and Hair Care & Nails

- L'Oréal Paris Elvive Dream Lengths Curls No Build-Up Micellar Shampoo, Sulfate-Free, Silicone-Free, Paraben-Free with Hyaluronic Acid and Castor Oil. Best for curly hair to coily hair, 16.9 fl oz
- https://a.co/d/2N0YnMS

Shea Whitney 15 New *INCREDIBLE* Ways to Use CASTOR OIL!
https://youtu.be/7areFk6qVZE?si=JTCabluNPjW89KjH

- Rollerball Applicators: https://urlgeni.us/amzn/cS5uX

Video Links - Belly Fat

Dr. Janine Bowring ND Melt Belly Fat with This Surprising Hack | Dr. Janine
https://youtu.be/cM8TbyYsoVw?si=Iiot2YL50ekHFwff

Video Links - Pain Reduction and Other Health Tips

Melissa Gallagher 20 SURPRISING Benefits of Castor Oil Pack Therapy | Castor Oil Uses for Wellness
https://youtu.be/Kl9Z4d0R6hw?si=6eB1r4UmQTadIJe3

Video Links - Eyes, Feet and Bumps, Oh My!

Shea Whitney I Used CASTOR OIL for 30 Days and THIS Happened!!!
https://youtu.be/t1r72bbfG10?si=SjeZVPAEVZVA2uL6

Dr. Kim D'Eramo Castor Oil-shocking change in my body!
https://youtu.be/3esR-7JfVeA?si=K-aQ5iBc5QPbYfJT

Liz Stylish and Grateful - Fashion over 40 SHOCKING Castor Oil results after 60 Days!
https://youtu.be/lDdsZ64gcWU?si=koKn6H1o6JdXL1YV

Video Links - Beyond the Body - Interesting Castor Oil Tips

Shea Whitney 15 New *INCREDIBLE* Ways to Use CASTOR OIL!
https://youtu.be/7areFk6qVZE?si=jSQBjcb81aPzCSZv

9

References

astel's Health Foods [Mastel's Health Foods Est. 1968]. (2014). UNVEILING THE ANCIENT ELIXIR: CASTOR OIL'S HISTORY AND MULTIFACETED USES. *Mastel's Health Foods,* https://www.google.com/search?q=UNVEILING+THE+ANCIENT+ELIXIR%3A+CASTOR+OIL%27S+HISTORY+AND+MULTIFACETED+USES&oq=UNVEILING+THE+ANCIENT+ELIXIR%3A+CASTOR+OIL%27S+HISTORY+AND+MULTIFACETED+USES&gs_lcrp=EgZjaHJvbWUqBggAEEUYOzIGCAAQRRg7MgYIARBFGDzSAQgxNDE4ajBqN6gCCLACAQ&sourceid=chrome&ie=UTF-8#vhid=zephyr:0 & vssid=atritem-https://www.mastels.com/blogs/news/unveiling-the-ancient-elixir-castor-oils-history-and-multifaceted-uses.

https://www.mastels.com/blogs/news/unveiling-the-ancient-elixir-castor-oils-history-and-multifaceted-uses

Curtis, L., & Bard, S., MD. (2023). Health Benefits of Castor Oil. *Health.* https://www.health.com/castor-oil-benefits-6827595

Alookaran, J., & Tripp, J. (2022). Castor Oil. *National Library of Medicine.* https://www.ncbi.nlm.nih.gov/books/NBK551626/#:~:text=Castor%20oil%20is%20most%20well,use%20as%20a%20stimulative%20laxative.

Qhemet Biologics. (n.d.). The history & benefits of castor oil. *Qhemet Biologics.* https://qhemetbiologics.com/blogs/news/the-history-benefits-of-castor-oil

Whitney, S. (2023, November 12). *I Used CASTOR OIL for 30 Days and THIS Happened!!!* [Video]. Shea Whitney Style. https://www.youtube.com/watch?v=t1r72bbfG10

Solar Girl Homestead. (2023, December 24). *Castor oil for your face | INCREASE Benefits by 3 TIMES | The right WAY to use it to* [Video]. https://youtu.be/U4tYTUxXPwQ?si=bh6CuXZ6XeMfr8eN

SolarGirl Homestead. (2023, May 29). *The Best Moisturizer: Removes Wrinkles, Scars, and gives Amazing Complexion* [Video]. https://youtu.be/NaVP7v5rM9Q?si=EdBzQlHTIWCL2-Vx

REFERENCES

Arbon, P. (n.d.). *Turbo Charge Your Castor Oil and Face Massage with Ice Water Dips Over 50* [Video]. https://youtu.be/ZRmpixiQ5Kc?si=0c9ky Y8MIsIz7d9t

Basile, L. M., MFA, & Robinson, M., MD MBA. (2023). What Is Gua Sha, and How Do You Use It to Sculpt Your Skin? *GoodRX Health.* https://www.goodrx.com/well-being/alternative-treatments/gua-sh a-facial-stone-benefits

Johnson, C. (2024, March 3). *Castor Oil Changed My Skin in 30 Days (SHOCKING RESULTS Over 50)* [Video]. https://youtu.be/rXvD2e_ FLhc?si=hJxCDci6iBVolJ8q

Anastasia, S. (2020, April 23). *https://youtu.be/J-jG2ZsqrG8?si=AbBebWg P1csRqbSs* [Video]. https://youtu.be/J-jG2ZsqrG8?si=pubTbHD3zjOp HLb0

Shillington, S., ND. (2020, January 17). *How castor oil can get rid of your acne.* [Video]. https://youtu.be/cK2wYh6a9Nk?si=5Y7J4_MwU3OU zhkA

Atkins, S. [Fabulous Over 50]. (2024, February 15). *My SHOCKING Castor Oil Results After 30 Days As a Woman Over 50* [Video]. https://yo utu.be/mhg86xl8v5Q?si=rt6s3xNJE3yLgNZj

Gallagher, M. (2023, May 1). *20 SURPRISING Benefits of Castor Oil Pack Therapy | Castor Oil Uses for Wellness* [Video]. https://youtu.be/Kl9Z4d0R6hw?si=P0JsbhcNDWZn5xHW

Whitney, S. (2024, May 22). *15 New *INCREDIBLE* Ways to Use CASTOR OIL!* [Video]. https://youtu.be/7areFk6qVZE?si=m1h0cK_e7_tLItIt

Roos, D. (n.d.). 5 Things You Didn't Know About Your Belly Button. *Howstuffworks.* https://health.howstuffworks.com/human-body/parts/5-things-didnt-know-about-belly-button.htm

Digestive System: Ileocecal Valve (ICV) Dysfunction. (n.d.). *The Hayden Institute.* https://haydeninstitute.com/specific-conditions/digestive-system-ileocecal-valve-icv-dysfunction

Bowring, J., ND [Dr Janine]. (2023, August 22). *Melt Belly Fat with This Surprising Hack | Dr. Janine* [Video]. https://youtu.be/cM8TbyYsoVw?si=3fV-AtOW9PxdKwF-

D'Eramo, K., D. O. (2024, January 29). *Castor Oil-shocking change in my body!* [Video]. https://youtu.be/3esR-7JfVeA?si=bjHnbiEpOy5Qop2A

REFERENCES

Stylish & Grateful [Fashion Over 40]. (2024, January 28). *⛩SHOCK-ING👀Castor Oil results after 60 Days!* [Video]. https://youtu.be/1DdsZ 64gcWU?si=uM86Kt_WXS_yXsk0

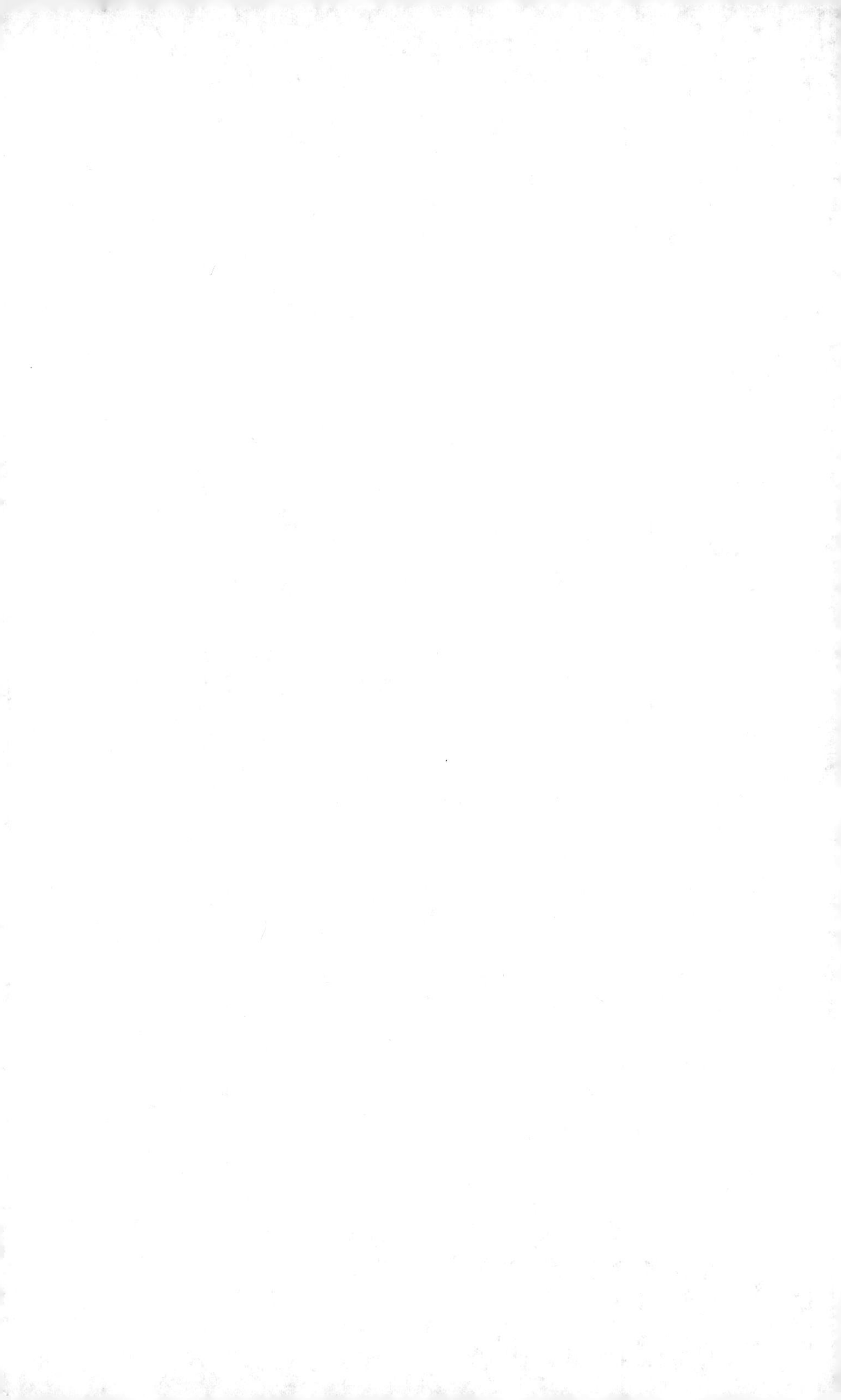

www.ingramcontent.com/pod-product-compliance
Lightning Source LLC
Chambersburg PA
CBHW051856250726

48659CB00006B/2248